Good End

End-of-Life Concerns and Conversations about Hospice and Palliative Care

with

Michael Appleton, MD

Good End: End-of-Life Concerns and Conversations about
Hospice and Palliative Care

Published by Hats Off Books®
610 East Delano Street, Suite 104
Tucson, Arizona 85705 U.S.A.
www.hatsoffbooks.com

Cover art by Michael Appleton.

Publisher's Cataloging-in-Publication
(Provided by Quality Books, Inc.)

Appleton, Michael, 1932-
    Good end : end-of-life concerns and conversations
about hospice and palliative care / with Michael
Appleton.
    p. cm.
    LCCN 2005925297
    ISBN 1-58736-481-6

    1. Terminal care. 2. Hospice care. 3. Palliative
treatment.   I. Title.

R726.8.A665 2005   362.17'5
                                QBI05-600025

Tell all the Truth but tell it slant—
Success in Circuit lies
Too bright for our infirm Delight
The Truth's superb Surprise
As Lightning to the Children eased
With explanation kind
The Truth must dazzle gradually
Or every man be blind

—Emily Dickinson

TO ANNA

Introduction

People have a great many concerns at the end of life. The prospect of dying can be overwhelming and it may be difficult to make decisions. Advice comes from many sources and it may be hard to understand all of the information you get. Your questions have been asked before, by others going through similar situations. It is important for those of us who care for patients at life's end to never forget that while many of the situations that arise may seem commonplace to us, they are new for you. There are new terms, new treatments, new drugs, and new worries at the worst time—when you're not feeling well. While the Internet is a valuable source of information, the volume of information and conflicting opinions may be unsettling and actually contribute to your stress. The rapid segue or uninterrupted transition from the time of diagnosis to the introduction of hospice care can be overwhelming, confusing, and feel unreal. All of your concerns should be addressed as you seek to make the best choices for the end of your life. There may be several answers to a single question and the best one may be the one that just feels right for you. It's important to respect and trust your gut feeling. All of us have what's called selective hearing and screened memory. We hear only parts of things said and remember only pieces of what we've heard. Things have to be repeated and it may take a while to understand. Here are some questions and some responses; the kind of conversation you and I might have if we were sitting together in your home. Some of the conversations are with patients and some are with family members and caregivers. These are all recreations of actual events.

The interchanges are intended to stimulate thought and address fears and worries. It can be helpful to provide some insights into why people behave as they do around death and dying but it is virtually impossible to address all issues and answer all questions. Hospice professionals may be able to better deal with specific issues. There are, however, many common themes and hopefully these discussions will be helpful.

This is a journey that does not need to be done alone.

Preface

I chose to indicate the main topic of each discussion in the table of contents, however some of the questions and responses are about more than one single topic. Many of the issues are related and an answer to one concern leads to another that also needs to be discussed. Important issues you've not yet considered may appear. It is for this reason that I hope you'll read as much as possible rather than limiting yourself to one particular topic. There is a common thread running through the book, which will become more obvious as you read through the conversations. It weaves a fabric of honesty, authenticity, bravery, some humor and, of course, love.

As human beings we can share our common flaws and imperfections as well as our potential for magnificence. This process begins with communication.

Table of Contents

#1 About hospice

My doctor referred me to a hospice. Just what does that mean and why do I have to go there? I'd rather stay at home.

Well, first of all, hospice isn't just a place. Hospices did begin as places where the sick could go to be taken care of at the end of life. There still are hospices where dying people can go for care. We think of hospice, really, as a particular kind of concept or philosophy of care at the end of life, where even when cure isn't possible, relief of pain and other symptoms is provided. Hospice is like the bond that can hold things together at the end of your life. It binds us to you and your loved ones. We become a part of a healing family to make your journey easier. Most hospice care is done in the home, so you don't have to go someplace else; relief happens where you live. I prefer to think of hospice as palliative care (providing comfort) with the emphasis on living as best you can in the time left rather than concentrating on death and dying. I know that's hard to do when you get bad news about a terminal diagnosis and all your care focuses on sickness rather than wellness. During the transition from aggressive curative treatment to hospice care with emphasis on relief it is often difficult to think of this confusing period as the beginning of an opportunity to focus on quality of life. It takes some time to adjust. Please let hospice help you along one day at a time.

#2 Hospice: the "H" word

Doesn't hospice mean I'm going to die soon? And if it doesn't and I live for six months, do I have to die on time, get kicked out, or what?

For most people "hospice" is a scary word. Yes, it is about dying, but more importantly—and I want you to listen carefully to this—hospice is about caring when cure is no longer possible. It's about living the best way you can during the end of your life. No, you are not required to meet some schedule for dying and it would be great if we could kick you out if you had some miraculous cure. Actually, I have never seen that happen. On occasion, some people improve for a while and may even decide to stop a hospice program. Our mission is to help you to live as fully as you can. Hospice care is always a choice and you can always change your mind. We will always be here if you need us. Hospice programs have unlimited benefit periods and we stay with you as long as you need us and want us. If I could give you any one piece of advice it would be to focus on living now, as well as you can.

I know I repeat myself when I talk about "the Now" but in truth it's the only place you can be and have any power. Let us help you and let us take care of the worry about tomorrow. As paradoxical as it seems, in this time of crisis, hospice can offer an opportunity. The reality that the end of life is in sight is often a stimulus for people to use this living time as the final stage of growth. It is here in hospice that you can find the guides to reach that goal.

#3 New advice

My doctor and the cancer specialist both explained
everything about my disease to me and I feel comfortable with what I'm doing. Now my sister comes
from back east and demands that I get another
opinion from a good doctor she's heard about who
has developed a new treatment that can cure my
cancer. What should I do?

My first response would be to tell you to tell your
sister to mind her own business and send her back east.
On second thought, maybe it would be best to understand
your sister's concerns. If she's like most people in this situation, she feels helpless and powerless and wants to do
something, anything, to help. She may feel some guilt for
not being as close to you as she thinks she should have
been. In any event, it's probably best to just sit with her,
explain everything, and even ask her to participate in a
meeting with your hospice team. She's no doubt worried
about losing you and this visit is really a wonderful
opportunity for you two to spend some time together. She
needs to be your sister and take care of you and you can
let her help; that's the gift you give to her.

It sounds as if you trust your physician and your
oncologist. I certainly believe in second opinions, but
there are situations where another piece of advice just
stirs up the pot, wasting money and living time. There
will always be news about dramatic cures. It's interesting
how so much of that information appears on the front
pages of the magazines and papers at the supermarket
checkout counter. Most of that stuff encourages false hope
and ultimately leads to disappointment. It stimulates
denial and the secret hope we all share that maybe a
miracle will occur. There are a lot of cracks in medicine—
fewer today than in the past, perhaps. Just the same, there

are still the snake-oil salesmen, promising to fill in the cracks—only now they're on TV and the Internet. Maybe it's best to trust the decisions you've made with your physician and get on with living.

#4 Morphine: the "M" word

The doctor wants to give me morphine for pain. Doesn't that mean I'm going to die soon? And I'm really afraid of getting addicted. Besides, I am definitely not a pill person!

Wow! Where have I heard that before? There are three parts to your question: morphine, addiction, and dying soon. Actually there is a fourth part that you slipped in at the end of the question: being a "pill person." Let me try to address all of your concerns.

First, any treatment begins with an explanation— especially treatment with morphine. Morphine is called "God's Medicine." It's a wonderful drug to relieve pain and it really helps with breathing difficulty. Morphine has some side effects and a lot of myths about it. The myths are just false notions or exaggerations. I tell patients that addicts use drugs to escape reality—people in pain use drugs (like morphine) to relieve pain so they can better experience reality. When the pain goes, the need for painkillers like morphine goes. In the old days, doctors reserved morphine until the end and in those days, before hospice and palliative care, people suffered needlessly. I can't see any benefit in suffering. If there are side effects from morphine, they usually disappear, and there are other drugs we can substitute if we have to switch. I don't recommend the needless use of any medication, but if you have pain, morphine is really effective.

Forget about addiction. If you need a medication for comfort, take it. And no, we don't save a good drug like morphine for "the end." In this century we use morphine early for one simple reason—it works. There is no upper limit to how much we can give as long as we increase it slowly and observe how much relief it allows. We give it early and use as much as is needed for as long as it's needed. The biggest problem with morphine, besides the myths, is that it causes constipation. That can be treated! Actually we want to treat constipation before it happens. Morphine is an opioid and a good piece of advice is "start an opioid, start a laxative." First and foremost, the use of morphine begins with an explanation.

As for you not being a pill person, I'm not sure what that means. No person was born to take medicine; however, medicines in the form of pills or vaccines have extended our life expectancy and markedly improved people's health. Yes! Some people take pills for any little thing and some doctors prescribe a lot of drugs. I think the important thing for you to remember is that taking pills does not mean you are a weakling or less of a person. Toughing it out and using willpower to heal isn't very helpful and usually doesn't work. That kind of stoic behavior will not earn you a medal for bravery. You may, however, get an award for being stubborn. If you have a life-limiting illness then obviously you will die at some future date. Using morphine does not mean death is near. Needless concerns about necessary medicines and their side effects is a way your mind keeps you from enjoying the present moment. Take the pills!

#5 Losing vigor

I'm not able to do all the things I used to do. I feel useless and I'm becoming a real burden to my family.

That's a very common complaint and it doesn't help for me to say, "Oh yes! I know just how you feel," because I really don't know. It also does not make you feel better if I tell you that most people in your condition feel that way. That kind of information feels dismissive. It doesn't help your suffering to know others are also suffering. What's needed here is a reality check and a shift of focus to what's good and can help. It doesn't do much good to dwell on things that can't be completely fixed or the things you can't do anymore.

Let's look at the situation from a different perspective. Some people refer to this as "reframing." Let's look at what can be done. There are some medicines that can help a lot. That's not the whole answer, but it's a hopeful start. A little bit later we can discuss other things that work.

The best medicine, I think, is not in a pill form. It's being able to sort out your feelings and talk with others about those things that are worrisome. Hospice counselors, who simply listen without dishing out platitudes, do a great job. Getting over a lot of this stuff can only be done by going through it with people who can act as guides in these difficult times. I visited an eighty-three-year-old woman today who started crying when I asked her how she felt about her illness. I simply asked, "What's going on inside?" She told me that she used to work three jobs and clean her house and pay all the bills. Now she can't do much at all without becoming short of breath and feeling very weak.

It was important for me to realize how much she believed her value as a human being was based upon her ability to do things. That was her sense of self and she was losing it. Not only did the loss cause her sadness, it left her feeling, "If I can't do the things that I think make me who I am, then who am I?" I tried to explain a few things to her but realized that first I needed to just hear her out. Listening to a story all the way through has a healing effect. Explanations are fine but sometimes we just need to get through the sadness before we can take in any information. Even when I simply explain things, some people who've spent a lifetime developing the idea of the person they are cannot grasp the idea of their value as a person apart from what they do and the things they have.

#6 Allergies and overdose

> I took morphine once and got sick. I have an allergy to morphine and don't want it. Besides, it is too strong and I am worried about taking an overdose of narcotics.

There's really been no documented allergy to morphine. What you probably mean is that it made you sleepy or nauseated. Those are side effects that usually go away after a few days. Sometimes morphine can cause itching, which can seem like an allergy. Morphine is similar to the body's own endorphins and an allergic reaction is unlikely. Occasionally morphine has been mixed with another substance, which caused an allergic response. Still, the bottom line is that if you are frightened or don't want to take morphine, don't. You shouldn't take any medication you don't want. There are other alternative opioids such as methadone, oxycodone, Dilaudid (hydromorphone), and Fentanyl. It might be easier to simply switch in the beginning if you are concerned.

As far as overdose is concerned, as long as you are still having pain, taking too much of an opioid such as morphine rarely causes an overdose. You'd be surprised at the large amounts of narcotics that are used to relieve pain and are still well tolerated. These drugs need to be increased slowly and carefully even though there is usually no definite upper limit. The majority of physicians are not familiar with the use of opioids for pain. Many pain specialists use highly technical injection devices to relieve pain. My experience is that the oral administration of pain medication is very effective in over 90 percent of patients. That's why you need to consult experienced hospice and palliative care specialists. It is important to sit down with your prescribing doctor and feel comfortable, trusting that you will obtain relief from the correct drug given to you.

#7 Suffering in silence

I have a high pain threshold and can take a lot of pain. I'm not that sick and I'm not a sissy.

Good. I'm glad you have the ability to tolerate pain. My advice is to take medication only if you want to be comfortable. A patient once told me that having pain let him know he was still alive. I really don't see the benefit of that attitude, however; suffering is optional and you know relief is available if you choose. Getting necessary pain relief does not make anybody a sissy. It simply takes the "bear it" out of "grin and bear it." The amount of pain you experience may not always be an indication of how sick you are. You get to choose how comfortable you want to be. If being tough is important to you, by all means go for it! I'd like to remind you that there is pain other than physical pain. Physical pain keeps you from totally getting on with activities of living. It is that underlying nagging discomfort that diverts you from talking about your feelings and managing unfinished business at the end of your life.

#8 Starvation and dehydration

We're worried about mom. She is not eating or drinking. She is going to starve to death and she's getting really dehydrated. She better get back to the hospital or at least get some IV fluid.

This is a very important concern. If mom has an end-stage disease and is getting worse from widespread cancer, feeding probably won't help. If this is the situation, food will not nourish her back to health. It may prolong the process of dying and the discomfort that goes with it. In cases like this feeding becomes an unnecessary burden when patients naturally lose their desire to eat. At the end of life, the purpose of food should be enjoyment, not nutrition. There are no strict rules about feeding and a lot depends upon the disease and the patient's desire or ability to eat and swallow. Certainly we would not feed a person who cannot swallow. We worry about people choking or aspirating food into their lungs, which can be a big problem. So why not stick a nasogastric tube into the stomach? Because it's uncomfortable. And a gastrostomy (a tube directly into the stomach through the belly wall) may prolong life but there are also complications. Ask yourself—is it worth it? For some persons it may be acceptable to be artificially fed. For others, it may not help the quality of their life.

Feeding is always a delicate issue because so much of eating is about giving and love and represents the way families communicate and share affection. Hydration is another touchy issue. Both starvation and dehydration are buzzwords that conjure up agonizing pictures of starving third-world children. Fluid and nourishment should be provided to people who have the capacity to recover, but when recovery is impossible we need to rethink the effects of our good intentions. People lose their appetites and the sense of thirst also diminishes. IV fluids can cause overload and congestion. Dry mouth can be relieved even when people can't swallow by using lemon-flavored swabs and providing good oral care.

There are some situations in which hydration with a subcutaneous (under the skin) infusion of fluid may relieve confusion or delirium. Thirst may not be relieved and often is not uncomfortable if there is good mouth care. It is unkind to ship a dying person off to the hospital for treatment. That's not a comfortable way to die. Much of the discomfort about not feeding and pushing fluids comes from the family and not the patient. The feeling of helplessness can be overwhelming and there often seems to be a sense of urgency about getting something done— anything! There is much that can be done for comfort at the end of life. Food and fluids are fairly far down on the list.

#9 Herbs and vitamins

> My father is dying of cancer. He doesn't eat much and seems to be withering away. I heard about some vitamins and herbal preparations that they sell. I want my dad to take them so he'll get stronger. He just looks so weak. I just don't know what to do.

I understand the feeling of not knowing what to do; the sense of powerlessness and helplessness is really hard to withstand. If your dad has a terminal illness and is dying, no amount of supplements will help. Any pill or supplement one takes may have what is referred to as a "placebo effect." If you take a substance and really believe that it will be beneficial—particularly if a lot of money was paid for it—you may feel better. If that provides comfort, it causes no harm, and the product is not used in place of current prescribed drugs, I see no harm except to your pocketbook. Those ads for healing cures are frequently deceiving and are designed to sell hope. Usually it's false hope and amounts to what we used to call a wallet-extraction procedure. You might feel better about having done something but I doubt if your father is going to benefit substantially. Here is where doing something is probably not of much value. It may be better to just spend time with your dad—being instead of doing.

At the risk of repeating myself, it's important to understand that medicine is full of cracks in our knowledge. The more we understand, the more cracks and imperfections there will be; more things to learn and understand. That doesn't mean we should abandon traditional medicine and throw the baby out with the bathwater. It also doesn't mean that some alternative therapies are useless. It simply means that you must be cautious and wary. There always seem to be people who appear with magical thinking and worthless mortar to fill those cracks. These people, usually untrained and full of anecdotes, profit from offering false hope in attractive packaging.

Contrary to some uninformed sources, I don't believe there is an organized conspiracy to keep people from receiving effective therapies. I believe organized medicine, although moving slowly and cautiously, is recognizing the value of complementary therapies and incorporating them. Actually, if you are truly interested in useful herbs, botanicals, and vitamins your best source would be a naturopathic physician (ND). Naturopaths are trained physicians skilled in prescribing natural substances correctly. In your particular case, giving another substance isn't going to help much. Your presence is the best medicine.

#10 Depression

My sister looks so sad and depressed since she found out she has cancer. She has lost weight and sleeps a lot more. Can we give her an antidepressant or something to pep her up and give her more energy?

People who are fatigued (which happens with most terminal illness) often look sad. Depression is a normal reaction to learning that your life will end. It never seems to be when you planned—if you truly ever did have a timetable. People go through many emotions when dealing with tragic and unanticipated events, particularly the prospect of dying.

Having to be with your sister at this difficult time is very hard to endure. Just be sure that you don't want to fix your sister so you don't have to tolerate her pain. Everybody wants to help, to fix things in some way. Being with a sad, withdrawn, depressed person is very challenging because the healing that you bring is not in the form of good advice or suggesting that your sister "cheer up." Your help is not necessarily with an antidepressant medication (which may be only part of the help). Your gift (and it is a gift) is your presence. When a person is faced with the end of their life they may experience several kinds of emotional reactions. This is the unpredictable human way of coping. It can be difficult to be around a person who is angry or withdrawn. Some people act as if their terminal diagnosis doesn't exist when it's clear that's not the case. Others desperately look for ways out of an inescapable end. Some people appear docile and accepting as if they are at complete peace with their situation or perhaps ignorant of what's going on. It is impossible to predict what behavior to expect and it's a challenge to know the optimum response. There may be times when you can't seem to get it right and when the best response may be no response. Your willingness to simply be present, there with your sister, without any expectations and without any sage advice, for however long it takes, is good therapy—for her and for you.

Depression is a state that is often difficult to describe to someone who has not experienced it. It is more than the feeling of sadness. Some people experience a sense of hopelessness along with an actual feeling of distress in the chest. Perhaps this is what has been described as heartache. In any event, the experience is that of being lost and sometimes thinking that nothing is right now, nor will it ever be right again. Severe depression requires medication. Treating with antidepressants cannot change reality but it can significantly alter perception, lift the cloud, and improve the quality of life. There are many drugs that are effective. This is a vital issue to be discussed with your hospice physician.

#11 Short of breath

> I am short of breath. The doctor said it's normal with my lung cancer. I am afraid I'll suffocate or choke to death at the end. I am so frightened.

I understand. I hear you.

The idea of being trapped in a horrible state of choking or smothering is very frightening. That is not happening now. With good care it will not happen. Your job is to stay present and let us manage problems in the future. There are many things that can happen with lung disease as it gets worse, but none of them are beyond effective treatment to keep you comfortable. Morphine, breathing assistance, sedation, and other therapies, provided by skilled and experienced (and caring) professionals, will not allow suffering. We usually do a good job of keeping our promises. People frequently want to know how long they have to live. It's very difficult to predict. Most of their worry is about experiencing pain or other overwhelming situations. Hospice people are trained to anticipate and avoid these problems. I know there is always an underlying fear of the unknown. If you realize most of that stuff is in your mind and not actual, you can tell your head-machine to shut up and you can bring your attention to the present moment. This present moment is a place where your mind can't be. It takes some practice but you can actually stay in the present. That's where your life is.

#12 Denial

> My husband is old but he usually has a good memory. I was in the room when the doctor told him he has cancer in several sites in his liver. He seems to not want to talk about his diagnosis and keeps referring to "those leavings in his liver" that his doctor talked about. What is going on?

I think the doctor said "lesions" in the liver and your husband heard "leavings."

Lesions are abnormal findings that are unclear, usually seen in a scan or x-ray, that are not specific. Frequently they are cancer and we (doctors) skid around saying cancer or malignancy by using words such as tumors, growths, spots, neoplasms, or lesions. If we avoid the difficult words, maybe we'll also be able to avoid discussing an uncomfortable subject in the moment—sort of "don't ask, don't tell." And actually we may really be uncertain and wish to avoid causing undue concern about something that may not be present—such as cancer.

If your husband was told he had cancer, using that exact word, his avoidance of the specific term is denial. It's the natural way we protect ourselves from an unpleasant reality. He probably knows and can't quite come to accept the diagnosis and its consequences yet. That's his choice. Most of that denial is active at a subconscious level for automatic self-protection. You don't have to force him to talk about cancer. It won't hurt him if you do use the word and you really don't need to protect him. Just don't beat him over the head with a reality he is not ready to accept. Do what you feel is most comfortable without causing unneeded stress. At some future time you'll probably need to discuss the reality of the diagnosis—whatever you choose to call it.

A bigger problem is if he has not been told. Withholding, or not telling the truth, is a covert way of lying. While it may be uncomfortable to disclose this important information, it deprives the person of making his own choices about how to live the rest of his life. If people don't want to know the unpleasant facts, they will not hear you because they have this built-in defense mechanism called denial. Telling the truth may be stressful for you in the moment; it will not cause suicidal depression or hasten death in the person who receives the information. Truth needs to be given—sometimes slowly, in pieces, and in a supportive way. Maybe your entire family needs to be involved to support you and the person who gets the news in the discussion process.

#13 Withholding

Grandma went to the doctor because she had some chest pain and weight loss. She's ninety-two and fairly alert. She always keeps busy cleaning her house and doing stuff. While she was getting dressed, after the exam, the doctor took us aside and told us she had far advanced breast cancer. He did not tell her because he said she was too old to do anything and telling her would only cause her to give up and die sooner. None of us know what to do.

This is a variety of the last question. Certainly if your grandma had dementia and couldn't understand, there'd be no value in telling her. It might cause some upset and should perhaps be left unsaid. My friend's mother has advanced dementia and when his father died, she missed him and knew he was gone but couldn't remember much more.

To keep telling her something painful that she couldn't comprehend and remember seemed cruel and unnecessary. I do not agree with the doctor's advice even though he knows her better than I. There are ways to gently bring up the subject by asking questions such as, "Do you want to know what the doctor said?" She probably knows somewhere inside herself. Give her the opportunity to ask. Sometimes worrying about the unknown can be worse than dealing with the known, because when it's out there and articulated she can deal with it if she chooses (which may include ignoring it).

#14 Do not resuscitate (DNR)

> My brother has had several heart attacks and a bypass graft. He takes a pile of medicines for his heart and his diabetes. His cardiologist told him that nothing more could be done for him and, on the way out of the exam room, mentioned that he was putting in a referral for hospice. I don't know what to do now. My friend told me that if my brother goes on hospice he has to sign a DNR so they won't revive him if there's an emergency.

I'm sorry your visit went that way. I won't apologize for the doctor. I know some physicians have a very difficult time with end-of-life issues and simply can't talk with patients about dying. There are many doctors who do spend time talking to their patients and families about these important issues. Let's try to clear up some of your concerns and discuss how you can assist in your brother's care and get the needed support.

Your brother obviously has advanced heart disease and has been through a great deal of tests and procedures, which have kept him alive. The operations themselves cause a great deal of physical stress and I'm sure your brother is on a pot-full of pills. There finally comes a time when there is just no more that can be done to repair a failing heart. The end of life can be made comfortable at home without resorting to calling paramedics and beginning uncomfortable procedures to save a heart that simply cannot be restored to a functional state. To begin CPR is to inflict pain at the end of life. This suffering is compounded by placing an endotracheal tube in the airway, inserting intravenous lines, and doing other life-saving measures, none of which will help much. A DNR, however, is not mandatory. You should definitely not be forced to sign such a document. You should freely choose to sign these papers, which are intended to prevent a futile and painful end to your brother's life. Ending up on a ventilator in an intensive care unit is not a pleasant experience for a patient or family. Hospice should be able to assist you in caring for your brother at home at the time of his death. At the end, avoiding a crisis that can disrupt a comfortable and peaceful death is a wise choice.

#15 Animals, children, and G tubes

My father has dementia. He had a stroke and now is back at home where our family is taking turns caring for him. He is paralyzed on his right side and can't speak. He can take small sips of liquid but can't eat. I can't tell if he recognizes us or even understands what we are saying. The cats and dogs jump up on the bed with him and our kids climb up to talk to "Poppa." I am not sure if that's OK. Also, one of the doctors we saw the last time we were in the emergency room said we should feed him with a G tube. We're not sure what the best thing to do is.

Your situation is not at all unusual for us in hospice and it is unique and special for you. If your father is on a home hospice program, which Medicare provides, you can get a great deal of guidance from the entire hospice team. There are lots of facts to consider here. First, how bad was your dad's dementia before the stroke and what was his quality of life as he defined it? Most people don't think to comment on that when they're feeling well. What were his wishes when he could make decisions and what would he have wanted at the end of his life? Did your dad have a durable power of attorney? I'm sure you'll discuss all of this with the social worker. The important thing is to represent your father and respect his wishes.

A G (gastrostomy) tube can prolong life. In some cases continued feeding can keep people alive for enjoyable and important activities. In other cases, keeping people alive can prolong suffering, decrease their quality of life, and set them up for other complications, such as bedsores or regurgitation of feedings into the airway and aspiration pneumonia. The complications resulting from prolonging the end of life may be much worse and discomforting than simply withholding feedings.

24

I think it's great in your home with the animals climbing on the bed. Animals seem to sense when things are happening and they frequently mobilize for support. I've had a few dogs growl at me when I try to examine a patient at home. Dogs can really be territorial and guard their owners; fortunately, I've never been bitten. It is certainly important to involve children. Dying is a natural part of life and depending on their age, their understanding and response differs. I think it's healthier to bring them in and not to exclude them as if something frightening is going on. As far as a G tube is concerned, that goes back to what we discussed in question #8.

Frequently, when a patient cannot communicate, loved ones and friends want to know if the person can hear and if they should talk to him or her. I think the best answer is to assume you can be heard and talk — talk a lot. Sing, play music, read stories, and keep the room bright. Remember that talking is also important for you as a part of closure and as a way to express your feelings: your sadness and your love. Recently, when a good friend of mine was near death, his grown son, his wife, and I climbed on the bed with him where he was snuggled with his two Siamese cats. We sang to him and told him how much we loved him. I know he felt our love. I initially had some doubts about the propriety of all of us grown-ups jumping onto the bed of a dying person, but we performed an act of love. There is a part of me that knows, in the context of human connection, it's permissible to be spontaneous and somewhat irreverent.

#16 Pain pills and overdose

My wife has terminal breast cancer. She has a lot of pain and a big load of every kind of pill you can imagine. She is in bed most of the time and pretty weak. I don't know how to sort out her medications, what's important and what's not. I've been giving her the pain pills. They help some but seem to make her sleepy. I don't want to put her in a coma or give her an overdose. What's your advice on this?

I can give you some advice, however I don't know the extent of your wife's cancer.

If it is spread (metastatic) it is important to know the extent and other organs involved (particularly brain, liver, and lungs). Sorting out medications and deciding on what medications are important and which ones are useless now is up to a physician who is familiar with your wife. Staying in bed longer and being fatigued may be a direct result of the tumor, or anemia, or high blood calcium, or other factors that need to be sorted out by a hospice physician or your oncologist. Pills that were preventive in nature, such as vitamins and cholesterol-lowering agents, probably can be stopped. Some blood pressure medications may need to be reevaluated and either tapered or stopped if they are not essential.

Some pain pills can cause drowsiness initially and sometimes after pain medication is given, people sleep more because they can now rest better—pain-free. Sometimes there is just no happy medium between sleepy and pain-free vs. wide-awake and hurting. What would you choose?

Overdose with opioids (narcotics) is often a worry and most people are terrified of doing something wrong or making a mistake. Most mistakes are harmless and rarely are severe errors made in treating pain. If a serious event

26

did occur, an important question to ask yourself is what was your intention? If your intention was well meaning, an adverse consequence should not engender guilt or remorse. Your intention was to help—not to cause harm.

Let me say a few words about narcotics at this point. For drugs such as morphine, there is no upper limit to how much can be used. People do develop a tolerance and require higher doses as time goes on. That does not automatically mean the disease is progressing. The total dose is not as much of a problem as the speed of increasing each dose. Nearly always, pain relief comes first after a dose and perhaps some drowsiness. Rarely does morphine cause respiratory depression and the slowing rate of breathing is a good indicator to follow. As long as there is pain, opioids should be given.

#17 The end of ALS and assisted suicide

> My husband has Lou Gehrig's disease (ALS). He is slowly getting weaker and we're really worried about what's going to happen when he can't move. How do you plan for these things? We really are frightened about him dying a horrible death. My husband talks about just ending it all. Can we find a doctor to administer a lethal injection or give us enough medicine for an overdose?

First, let me say that I understand your fear. So much of fear is about unknown future events and not being able to be in control. Understanding more about what kind of decline you'll need to cope with will help. Please remember that you and your husband do not have to do this alone. I know you'll probably worry anyway, but please know that future concerns take up precious living time and keep you from enjoying what is available in the moment.

ALS is a particularly difficult disease because the mind is alert, the brain is functioning, and the patient is observing and experiencing the progressive loss of control of all of the body's muscles. Obviously this affects not only muscles of the arms, neck, and legs but eventually muscles controlling swallowing and breathing. The feeling of powerlessness, helplessness, and utter despair can be overwhelming. Many of the things we talk about may apply to other neurological diseases as well. Fortunately there is usually time to adjust to a decline in muscle strength. A hospice program can assist you both through your husband's illness. There are resources for patients with neuromuscular diseases and helpful advice is available. All advice must take into account your partic-

28

ular situation: your disease and its stage. Some recommendations for treatments and devices by well-meaning people stir up false hope followed by disappointment. In desperation, it is easy to grasp at straws and fall prey to nonmedical advice by persons offering treatments—often with ulterior motives. I say this not to discourage you, but to prevent you from becoming victimized by false hope.

As your husband becomes weaker and more dependent, moving from crutches to a walker to a wheelchair and finally to being confined to bed is a usual progression. Each change is usually met with some resistance, denial of what's apparent, anger, depression, and sadness. Expect it and ask for the support you need in moving through each decline. My experience is that most patients and families exhibit uncommon bravery in these situations. If you love your husband, please assure him that he is not a burden and that he presents you with a gift by allowing you to care for him. These can be both intimate and challenging moments. I'm also referring to bladder and bowel incontinence and diapers (which can be embarrassing).

Many problems such as stiffness of joints or your husband's inability to use his hands to eat or turn the pages of a book can be managed. The major problems we will face later will be those of speaking, eating, drinking, and breathing. I say "we" because we in palliative care will be there as your support system. These problems can be managed at home, but considerable thought must be given to these issues ahead of time with mutual understanding and agreements that respect your husband's wishes. At the end of life, each person must decide when there is not enough quality to continue with measures that maintain life. Artificial feeding by gastrostomy or nasogastric tube maintains existence but may not bring quality. Breathing machines, respirators attached to a tracheostomy, keep people alive and prolong the process of dying. Once started, they can be stopped later and the question that must be asked is, "Is the discomfort of a procedure and its possible complications worth the short-term benefit?" Stopping feeding when your husband cannot swallow is not uncomfortable and restricting fluid is not painful. Choking is preventable and suffocation, while a frightening thought to consider, will not be allowed with proper breathing support.

Without going into more detail I mention these situations, not to frighten you but to assure you that the end of life can be painless, peaceful, and comfortable. The mission of hospice is to make these promises come true.

You ask about assisted suicide. Suicide is the act of taking of one's own life. I have a problem with this act because of the wreckage it leaves behind. The survivors are invariably stunned and left wondering why the victim did not confide in them and ask for help. Suicide itself is nearly always an angry act and very often the survivors are left with their own unresolved anger. I understand that there are people who choose to end their own lives because of depression, their sense of hopelessness, or the belief that there is no other possible escape. It is really a sad situation when the mind ends up killing the body.

There are many excellent books written about this subject and I'd like to limit the discussion here to euthanasia, mercy killing and physician-assisted suicide. There are opposing thoughts about this act. As a physician with years of experience with the dying I have seen people who want their lives ended. I've also asked some of these people what it would take to change their mind. Often it is simply better pain and symptom control. In some instances a person will abandon the thought of prematurely ending his or her life if there is reassurance that the end will be made comfortable. I also have chosen not to be the appointed executioner for a patient who wishes assisted suicide. I'm not trained or comfortable doing this and I personally am not able to rationalize this as a benevolent deed.

I see other viable alternatives to killing the disease by killing the person who harbors the terminal disease. I also believe the active taking of your own life or choosing another to commit the act is a personal choice and ought not to be legislated—neither condoned nor forbidden. I realize there are places where the law allows such acts. This is one alternative. In most states, assisted suicide is still murder, whatever the compassionate intent. I've also seen circumstances where the family wants the patient's life terminated to stop their own anguish. Most people will not admit to this thinking but it is not an uncommon situation. There are times when suffering at the end of life can be prevented in a hospice setting with "palliative sedation" (rendering the patient unconscious until death occurs naturally). Here, the intention is not to kill, but to prevent any suffering until life ends.

I do not oppose assisted suicide on religious grounds. I recognize that this may be a major consideration for some people and I respect that. My experience has been that skilled hospice/palliative care physicians can manage pain and symptoms at life's end and if a lethal dose of a medication is given to relieve suffering and it results in death, the intention was to palliate and not to kill. Before you or your husband choose an act to end his life, please give it a great deal of consideration.

#18 AIDS—stopping therapy

My partner has been HIV-positive for five years and now has full-blown AIDS. He was doing well on his drug program but now he has drug side effects, more infections, and is losing weight. He is confused on occasion and his doctor says his viral load remains high and his lymphocyte numbers are going down. He does not want to stop his medication and refuses to sign a DNR form. If he gets worse, he wants to be taken back to the hospital. We've always wanted to be together at home at the end but he seems to have changed his mind.

While AIDS remains a life-limiting illness, treatments in the last two decades have improved the prognosis and allowed persons with the disease to experience a much better quality of life than previously. However, people still die of AIDS, and drug regimens are not always successful. Because people do improve with therapy and because so many of them are young, succumbing to the disease or the infections and other complications of the disease is a very hard reality with which to cope. It is especially hard when people with the disease who may have responded in the beginning later develop serious side effects from the drugs or fail to improve despite strict adherence to the treatment. It's even harder when the virus affects the brain and encephalopathy occurs. Intellectual function can deteriorate, judgment can be affected, and an actual state of dementia with delirium can occur.

Some of this may be happening to your companion. If his disease is progressing despite his therapy, there seems to be no value in continuing, particularly if he is wasting and has a diminished quality of life. Actually, he may feel better for a while if he is off of his medications near the end of his life. You, as his companion, may need to make some of the decisions for him. It would be very important to have it explained to you in detail just what going back to the hospital would entail, including the exact process of resuscitation.

People have the right to have CPR and lifesaving measures. They also must understand what happens with all emergency procedures. I doubt if your partner wants to go through a very painful and traumatic experience at the end of his life—from a disease where recovery is not possible. This is where the support of a hospice team and people from the AIDS community can provide expertise, directing your companion towards a better end-of-life outcome.

#19 Chemotherapy

> My mother is seventy-six years old and just came back from the hospital where she was diagnosed with lung cancer. The oncologist said that some chemotherapy might help. I'm not sure we should proceed with this. I've heard such bad things about chemo.

Age really shouldn't be a deciding factor, and seventy-six is not old. I don't know enough to give any specific advice. It's important to trust your physicians and ask the right questions in order to make the best decisions. Any decision should be your mother's although you certainly can have an influence and help guide her.

There are several kinds of lung cancer and treatments vary. If this is a primary tumor in the lung and not spread from elsewhere, you want to know about biopsy results, types of treatment possible, and the side effects of treatment. Because I don't know all of the facts I can't be specific and I don't want to guess. Chemotherapy can be beneficial and should be considered if your oncologist recommends it. In recent years oncologists have referred to some types of chemotherapy as palliative. This should mean that the benefits outweigh the risks, the side effects are usually mild, and life with quality can be significantly prolonged.

Some chemotherapy regimens may reduce tumor growth, slow a malignant disease process, and prolong life while also producing toxic side effects that also require additional treatment. Some questions to ask are: will this treatment cure her lung cancer and if not, will she live longer and comfortably?

When a statement is made such as "This may offer some benefit" or "This drug can be used here and may be worth a try," many people hear "cure" when none was offered.

It is necessary to ask about how much longer she can live with quality. If it's only a month or two statistically, is the treatment worth it and what are the side effects? What's the downside? What other treatments are available?

If you are satisfied with your advice, move forward with the knowledge that you made the best choice. Remember also that some people choose to have no treatment. Many hospice programs include radiation and chemotherapy as a part of their service in order to enroll patients sooner and provide support at the end of oncologic treatment. Perhaps it bears repeating that hospice should neither prolong the dying process nor hasten death. When cure is not possible and any treatment is diminishing the quality of life it should probably be discontinued. Obviously, this cannot be an absolute since each situation is different.

#20 Involving children

My wife is forty-four and is dying of stomach cancer. We have three children. Our youngest is a three-year-old boy. Our girls are six and ten years old. They know Mommy is very sick and stays in bed a lot. We don't want to go back to the hospital and have signed up with hospice so we can stay at home. I am so worried about the kids and don't know what to tell them.

I'm glad you called hospice. You and your wife and children should not have to go through this alone. It's so important that the children be involved, with you, at the end of life for your wife and their mother. Hospice counselors can help a lot. Often children are excluded from dying in a family situation and develop fear about a natural part of life. Children have different concepts of death and impermanence than adults depending upon their age. I could tell you about a few responses and behaviors to expect from your children; however, this is where professional assistance from experienced therapists is required. Kids act out their feelings and your being understanding and supportive toward their special way of grieving is essential.

#21 Helplessness and lack of control

My husband and I have been married for fifty-three years. He was just diagnosed with widespread cancer. After the biopsies and everything the oncologist said that there was nothing more that could be done and the social worker made a referral to hospice.

When my oldest son found out he went nuts and began bringing vitamins and health foods for his dad to eat. He seems angry because he seems to think we're not doing enough. We tried to contact our other sons but we haven't seen them in a long time and they have not returned our calls. Besides that, my sister is butting in and insisting we keep records of all of his medicines and when he takes them. She is always organizing things and making new lists. My husband is Catholic and his sister thinks it will help if he goes to church more even though he does not feel like it. This is a mess.

My first question is, "How do you feel?" It is so important that you take care of yourself and not be distracted by having to worry about taking care of the entire family's problems. Perhaps you need to take control of the situation and set things up the way you want them to be. It may be helpful to understand the behaviors of your sister and your son, but in the end they need direction and to be able to work through their own issues about loss without taking you and your husband hostage. Helplessness is manifested in many ways. People make lists and organize activities as a way of dealing with feeling out of control. Being angry and acting out is one way to channel suffering but it usually doesn't help, pushes people away, and shifts attention to the person who is angry. Dying brings out both the best and the worst behaviors in people.

Guilty people try to do something, anything, to relieve their sense of guilt. Structure needs to be established to stabilize the situation. Here is where the entire hospice team can come together with you, providing support for you and your family. Although your situation may have some moments of discomfort, it sounds like a lot less of a mess than you describe. Perhaps you can enroll your son in trying to contact his brothers. It would be helpful to get in touch with the hospice spiritual advisor (chaplain). This is the time to be strong and decisive. Focus on what can be accomplished rather than on what's not working and take charge.

#22 Coma

My nineteen-year-old son was injured in a car accident six weeks ago and is in a semi-coma. He doesn't open his eyes. He can't move or speak. He is being fed with a tube from his nose into his stomach. His doctor does not think he will recover or ever really wake up. He has suggested a feeding tube (gastrostomy) to keep him alive so we can take him home. My wife sits at his bedside and talks to him. She swears he hears her but I really don't see any response. I don't know what to do.

The first thing is not to make any decisions on your own. Any choices should be made carefully and with consultation. I'm sure you've had neurological consultation and there's nothing wrong with obtaining another opinion. There are situations in which people who were thought to be brain-dead have awakened, although I think that's rare. It is important to not give up hope for recovery without sufficient time. Perhaps a feeding gastrostomy will allow you to take him home in a home hospice program and get the support you need while deciding if and when to stop feedings and allow him to die at home. Again, this is not something you should do alone. Letting go is a process and if your son is not going to awaken, it may take some time for you to accept that his life is at an end. Accepting the death of any loved one is hard; particularly when it is your own flesh and blood. It's part of your own genetic material and a part of your life you are losing. There seems to be an unwritten belief that we are always responsible for our children and if they die, somehow we are negligent, at fault, or guilty. While this is usually not the case, many people feel that way and need to understand that it is as if our children are given to us on loan and at some time we need to release them. That may be easy for me to say and I truly understand how difficult that is to do. Part of the closure for you and your wife is to lovingly care for your child, hold him, sing to him, cry with him, and know in your heart that you did everything that was possible.

#23 Alone or lonely

When my doctor referred me to hospice I was happy
to have some help at home. I was feeling weak after
leaving the hospital. I'm feeling better now and
wonder if I really need to take all of these pills every
day. The nurses and the home health aides are nice
and so are the other people who visit but, you know,
every time they call or come by they concentrate on
my pain and keep reminding me that I'm sicker than
I feel and need help. Some of the people treat me like
a baby and sometimes they seem too busy to listen. I
like the help but there are times when I'd just like to
be left alone.

I guess we really do concentrate on your problems and
look for what's not working.

In our effort to help, we sometimes seem to pay more
attention to our agenda rather than yours. I guess it's
impossible for us not to be reminders of your sickness and
your dying and I think our focus should be on maintain-
ing your wellness rather than fixing your sickness. Even
our questions, like "Are you having any pain?" brings
pain to mind. Maybe we ought to ask, "Are you comfortable and what do you need?" We don't want you to be
lonely and yet you need to remind us when we are
encroaching on your solitude and privacy. Sometimes we
try to help too much and need to give you some breathing
space. I think our job is to be with you in the way you
want and your job is to tell us.

#24 Dying and addiction

My brother Fred and I live together. Fred was a heroin addict and an alcoholic. He has been clean and sober for fifteen years. I am also in recovery and was once married to an alcoholic. I work a good Alanon program which helped me a lot when I stopped my own drinking, went to AA, and finally got a divorce. Fred and I go to meetings together and life was good until he got sick with cancer of the liver. When a liver transplant was out of the question, Fred's doctor referred us to hospice. Fred was doing well and avoided taking anything for pain even though there was morphine in the house in case it was needed. Recently Fred has complained of some pain and has started taking a lot of morphine. The doctor isn't sure if Fred has as much pain as he says and is concerned that he's just using morphine to knock himself out at the end of life. Fred talks a little about dying but he spends most of his time looking confused, sleepy, and acting as if he were "drugged out." It's really hard to be around him when he acts inebriated.

This is a difficult situation that does not have a right answer. First, Fred has an addiction. Any addiction is a way to escape feeling feelings and certainly his liver disease is something from which he can't escape or recover. Fear and hopelessness can certainly cause him to withdraw. Hopefully the hospice social worker can become involved. Your question is whether he's using the morphine to get high and escape from the emotional pain of dying or because he is actually having physical pain. One would hope he knows why he's doping himself but maybe he doesn't. The stimulus behind reactivating an addiction is not always understandable. It would be important to understand so you could help.

Second, his liver disease may be causing some of the confusion and you should seek advice from his physician. There are medications that might reduce blood ammonia, if that's what is causing the confusion, and might clear him up a bit.

Third, once he has reactivated his addictive process, it may be impossible for him to stop using. Certainly the hospice people want to help him and do not intentionally enable his addiction. We are caught in a double bind in a situation like this.

Fourth, the behavior he shows from the morphine is similar to that of an alcoholic who is inebriated. It's not easy to be around that behavior and it may be reactivating for you in your own recovery process. He may be lonely and need you close. He may not know how to ask for intimacy and his using drugs may have the effect of pushing you away. You might explain some of this to him at a moment when he is lucid, but in the end, it's your choice how much closeness you can tolerate, under the circumstances, and when you need to distance yourself. Ultimately, it is his choice about how he wants his life to end.

If the situation were reversed you might behave differently. It's important to remember to just do the best you can at this difficult time, to take care of yourself, and to forgive yourself if things don't go as perfectly as you would wish. Remember also that you can't expect someone to die your death for you. By that I mean that we can all visualize the way we wish the end could be and sometimes the ending is just not ideal. Hospice and your friends from the twelve-step program should be able to help you through this difficult time.

The issue of addiction comes up in addicts and alcoholics who have terminal diseases other than liver disease. Many are reluctant to take narcotics for fear of relapse. Pain requires treatment. The problem with treating pain in a chemically dependent person is that the addiction can be reactivated by introducing an opioid or a substance that affects mood. People who are familiar with addiction understand that reactivating the underlying addiction is as if the disease is in the gym next door—always working out—and ready to reenter once the door is opened. Addicts can be clever and manipulate physicians while their disease is being fueled by well-meaning providers. When a person has a documented life-limiting terminal illness pain must be controlled, and if narcotics are used to control the pain they must be tightly monitored. It is easy for an addict-in-disease to charm and manipulate compassionate hospice personnel. In the end, the addict can choose how he or she wants to spend the final days of life: sober or drugged. I personally cannot dictate the quality of life I would choose for a patient. I can, however, choose not to become an enabler or have my compassion abused.

#25 Caregiver distress

My sister is a nut. I know that's not kind to say but her behavior has just gone ballistic since our mother was diagnosed with cancer. My mother does not know she has cancer. She's eighty-eight and just went to the hospital through the emergency room for the fifth time. My sister has power of attorney (if you can believe that) and takes her in to the hospital for any little thing. The last admission was for pneumonia on top of her emphysema. That was when blood in her urine was discovered, studies were done, and they found cancer all over her abdomen on a CT scan. The doctors advised my sister to put mom on a hospice program and stop trying to fix every unfixable thing in an old lady at the end of life. My mom refused a biopsy of her stomach and will not sign a DNR order.

My sister is the problem. She refuses any treatments offered and then turns around demanding Mom gets all kinds of tests. She refuses to have the words "hospice" or "cancer" mentioned in front of our mother and argues with every person hospice sends to help. She did sign on to hospice but still wants everything done to cure any small or large problem that arises. She is angry about everything the doctors missed and yet has prevented them from finding or treating the problems for which she seeks attention.

While this is a difficult problem it's unfortunately not unusual. Perhaps I should say that it is a frequent problem. Some people come unglued at this very stressful time, particularly if they have underlying psychological problems with fragile coping skills.

If your sister is emotionally troubled or really incapable of acting as the power of attorney, this may be an overwhelming challenge for her and perhaps you should obtain psychological help for her in addition to legal assistance in changing the power of attorney to a more stable person. I think the hospice personnel can assist you with sorting this out. If your sister is just very anxious and overwhelmed, hospice can also help to provide support and structure. This will help your sister through a situation where many caregivers feel insecure, helpless, frightened, and worried about making a mistake.

Trips to the emergency room can usually be avoided if a system is in place that guides her through the process of your mother's dying. Sometimes dying at home is not possible and an inpatient facility may be required. Your sister needs to trust that on some level your mother really is aware of what's happening and may actually be relieved to have the truth out in the open. The reality is usually better than the fear of not knowing and speculating. There are gentle ways of telling your mom and you should realize that if your mother does not want to hear the truth, her own protective denial system will enable her not to hear what may be unacceptable information in the moment. It would be totally inappropriate to assault her with information about cancer and death. It is vitally important to gently move forward in a stepwise fashion by asking what she knows, what she wants to know, and just how frank and honest she wants you to be. The truth sometimes needs to seep in gradually to be comfortably integrated in the mind.

As far as the DNR (do not resuscitate) is concerned, nobody can hold your mother hostage and force her to abandon what she believes to be lifesaving measures. The entire process of CPR and all of the invasive emergency activities, including IVs, intubation, ventilators, and life support activities should be explained to her factually and graphically. It is only then, with compassionate support from the hospice team, that she can choose to embrace a palliative and less traumatic ending.

#26 The house call

Hi, I'm Doctor Appleton. I'm here to check you over and answer any questions you have.

Boy! I must be pretty sick if they send a doctor to my house to check on me.

That's what I want to discuss with you. Your wife asked me to talk with you. But first I need to know what you understand about your sickness and just how open and honest you want me to be. Tell me what you know.

Well, I was feeling kind of weak and tired and the doctor put me in the hospital because I was anemic. They ran some tests and x-rays and told me I had this problem in my stomach.

Just what kind of problem did they say it was?

Some sort of growth.

Did they say it was cancer?

I think so.

So if it is cancer, did they want to do any surgery to cure it?

No, because they said it couldn't be cured and the doctor asked me if I wanted chemotherapy. I told them if it couldn't be cured, what was chemotherapy going to do?

And what did they say?

They said that it might get a little better or help some. They didn't sound too optimistic so I said no. And then they said that they would refer me to hospice and I should get my affairs in order. And that's it.

So how did you feel about all of that?

It sure didn't feel too nice or hopeful. It's like they're sending me home to die. Isn't that why you're here? Doesn't it mean I don't have much time left?

OK. Let's slow down a little and talk about this one step at a time. First of all, hospice is about taking care of people at the end of life and keeping them comfortable. This does not mean you are going to die immediately. Are you with me? Sometimes it's impossible to predict how long you've got and even though there may not be hope for living a long time I think our interest should be about how well you live now— today. Does that make sense?

Oh sure, it makes sense, and I'm glad you put it that way. I'm just worried about my wife and how she'll manage when I'm gone. Even now when I'm weak like this she has to do so much to take care of me. I'm really worried about her.

I hear you. That's why we're here. We're here to help both you and your wife. I need you to know to that while we can't cure your cancer, we can care for you and keep you comfortable. This is about making it easier for both of you. Look, why don't we get your wife in here while we're talking about this? I'm not comfortable leaving her out and it's really important to have you both involved in this discussion. How's that?

Sure. Why don't you call her in here? I'm just worried that we shouldn't talk too much about dying. She may not be able to take it. She's a real worrier.

You know, that's just what she said about you. She was afraid that if you knew how bad things were that you'd give up and die sooner.

That's pretty silly. I've always been tough. Why don't you bring her in here?

Now that we're here together and you both know that we're talking about cancer and end-of-life care, let me talk with you about our hospice team and what we do. The main thing is for us all to be together in this. We don't have to discuss everything at once; in fact I think I've said a lot at this visit. What is important is that you know that you're not alone here and we'll help you get through this. We want to make this whole time easier and manageable for you. I think you'll be surprised how well you'll both meet the challenges.

#27 Predicting the end

(Frequently at the end of a visit, the primary caregiver takes me outside, closes the door, and engages me in a soft-spoken conversation.)

Listen, Doctor! How long do you really think she's going to last?

I know you're concerned and have to make plans, but...

No, no, it's not that but her family wants to know when they should come for a last visit.

I'm a little uncomfortable talking in hushed voices away from a patient since the patient usually suspects some dark secret and feels excluded. In this case, I think it's all right since she's sleeping. Let me just say this: It's very difficult for us, as doctors, to be exact about how long a person will live. Studies have shown that we usually overestimate prognosis. She hasn't been eating much for about a week and I would guess maybe you've got a week or less. Please don't hold me to it.

But look — the question behind "How long?" is usually "How is it going to go at the end?" or "Will we be able to control things?" In almost all cases, such as this, it's not frightening and the end is peaceful. No big explosive or unmanageable event occurs. I don't think that's a worry. We usually can anticipate any problems and can be here with you to guide you. As far as the right time for family and friends to visit, the answer is almost always now. Let people know that they should come as soon as possible to say goodbye. It's better than arriving too late and this advice takes the responsibility off you. Let them make their own decision.

#28 Worries about the end

Doctor! Tell me exactly what the process will be like.

You're asking about the dying process?

Of course. I want to know exactly how it's going to be when I am dying.

I don't want to seem evasive and I can only tell you what I know from seeing people die, but since I haven't died I can only guess what it might feel like inside. I see people who become weak and drowsy. I see people whose pain and symptoms are relieved. People lose their appetite and usually their thirst. They sleep more and when the body shuts down the heartbeat stops and then the breathing slows down and stops.

I think it will be a peaceful and pleasant experience and it might help you to imagine going to a nice place.

Well, that sounds real nice and sweet but I'm sixty years old and I have ALS. Don't you think that's probably a hell of a lot different from some old geezer who conks out from a stroke or a heart attack and just bows out immediately? I'll bet there are some folks who really suffer when they die. Right?

You bet it's different from dropping from some sudden event. And sure; there are times when suffering does happen. You know as well as I that there are no guarantees about what your end of life will be like. Hospice usually succeeds in preventing an uncomfortable passing. I'll give you a blow-by-blow scenario of what might happen if you want. I think it's a waste of time to speculate and besides I don't have a crystal ball. My main concern here is not so much about the facts but about the fear and worry my discussion will create.

Looking forward to end-of-life events not only creates undue fear but it uses up precious living time—and your mind will keep jumping back to the bad stuff.

Some of the things I might describe won't even happen and, as you know from other challenging events in your life, the anticipation is almost always worse than the actual experience of going through the event itself.

Look! I'm not a baby and I'd rather get an idea of what to expect not only for me but for my family.

I understand completely, so let me run through the changes with you, understanding that I may exaggerate some difficulties and even mention things that will never come to pass. ALS is particularly difficult because, as the body weakens, the mind stays alert. Patients I've spoken to who have had the disease say it's like being trapped or locked in, eventually being wide awake and unable to move. Depending on what nerves are involved, talking may later become impossible. Early on in the disease, there is muscle weakness; in the arms and legs, usually. The weakness progresses and the inability to use the extremities means slowly graduating from a cane to a walker to becoming bedbound. At some stage you will need complete assistance with bodily functions and you may need diapers and a urinary catheter. You'll require help with eating. When swallowing becomes impaired, it is necessary to stop the usual feedings and consider having a tube inserted from your nose into your stomach (nasogastric), or having a tube placed directly into your stomach for feeding.

All of these life-prolonging efforts have side effects. You may also choose to simply stop eating. These are difficult decisions to make and really depend upon *your determination about the quality of your life and how long you wish to remain in a paralyzed state. Starvation and dehydration are unpleasant words and need not cause you discomfort as your condition declines. As the process continues, breathing may become more difficult and there are artificial means to continue ventilation and keep you alive. In my experience, the complications of prolonging life artificially are usually more uncomfortable than simply not beginning them in the first place. As the depth of breathing becomes limited, the lungs can continue to receive oxygen, which is provided by a mask or nasal prongs. The lungs however, retain carbon dioxide and eventually the high level causes drowsiness (also called CO_2 narcosis). Then, as you slip into a coma, your breathing will stop. Then your heart will stop and you will die. What I'm describing is not a painful or agonizing process. It is usually a quiet and gentle ending. Although I prefer not to go into these morbid details, I trust my description will be comforting in some way. Again, it's important to remember that choking, smothering, starving, and dehydrating are things that can be avoided.*

These are terrifying terms for preventable experiences—the end of life can made be painless and comfortable. This is what hospice is all about.

Another concern, about which you did not ask, is about the amount of care and attention you'll require. I frequently ask patients if they feel as if they are a burden for their family. Invariably, the answer is yes. I need to clearly affirm that you give those who love you a gift when you allow them to care for you. It is extremely important to remember this.

53

#29 Talking to the dying

Dad is just lying here and he opens his eyes a little but doesn't seem to respond. Even when we turn him he doesn't move. We stroke his head and talk to him but we don't know whether he can hear us or not.

When people are nearing the end of life and slip into a coma it's uncertain if they can hear and, even if they do, that they can understand. I trust that there is a possibility that something gets through and for that reason I encourage you to talk to him and comfort him. Saying things that you want him to hear is part of his closure as well as yours. These can be poignant shared moments for you and your family.

I once asked Elisabeth Kubler-Ross, who was a pioneer in the hospice movement in America, if she really could communicate with people in a coma. She claimed that she could. She also claimed that she had her own spirit guides. I doubted that. When I asked her how she could be so sure about these things, she looked at me sternly and said, "Oh Michael, you need to get rid of your negativity." I've spoken to people who see auras, have out-of-body experiences, and believe in supernatural phenomena, which all seem strange to me. Perhaps it's my pessimism that gets in the way of my having new experiences. People believe in a lot of things that can't always be validated scientifically. If having those beliefs does no harm and improves quality of life, I think that's valuable.

That's all kind of a long way of saying, "Talk to your dad." Don't whisper, and assume that when you speak your voice is heard.

#30 Changes in breathing

I know my friend is dying. She just lies there and I can't awaken her. She does not seem to be in pain but her breathing is funny. All of a sudden she stops breathing and I think it's the end and then she starts again. She breathes faster and deeper and then stops. How long can this go on and what's going to happen?

This is a hard situation to just sit with. There are no exact answers to how long this will take without knowing more specific information. Perhaps I can explain a few things to help you feel more comfortable. When the breathing center in the brain (medulla) is depressed at life's end, it becomes less sensitive to carbon dioxide for stimulation and breathing will stop until the carbon dioxide builds up again in the lungs and brain. Then the breathing resumes, blows off the carbon dioxide, and the cycle starts over again. This is called periodic or Cheyne-Stokes breathing. Later on when there is severe depression, the deep breathing ceases. There is no way to know just how long this will last, however it is frequently observed very close to the end.

This can be followed by labored breathing where the chest doesn't move as much and it appears that there is some struggling to breathe. It may appear as a gasping effort using the neck muscles. It is not experienced as suffering by the patient, who is unconscious. Sometimes there is noisy breathing and a gurgling sound in the airway (unfortunately called the "death rattle"). These events may not always occur and if they do, they are not a cause of distress for the patient. The sight and sound of these agonal events that appear as struggling are not causing pain to the patient but are very disturbing to be with.

There are some medications that can be used to dry the airway to stop the gurgling sound. Hopefully, most symptoms will be managed.

As difficult as this picture may seem, the actual process is tolerable. When that event occurs it's a time to hold your friend, who is leaving life, in just the same way as you would cradle a newborn who is crying as it enters life. Let me repeat that you do not have to do this alone. Hospice will remain with you and guide you.

#31 Doing more

You've examined my husband John and you've
looked at the records. It took them a long time to find
his liver cancer and when they did they said it was
widespread and couldn't be removed. This all has
happened so fast. I am really angry that it wasn't
found and fixed sooner. The cancer specialist said
that my husband would be made worse with
chemotherapy, so it wasn't done. When he became
jaundiced they did some stents in the liver but now
he's getting worse again. He is so yellow and so weak
and he sleeps a lot. Why can't they unclog those
stents so he'll get better again?

I am going to try my best to answer your questions.
You sound frustrated and angry. I am not going to patron-
ize you or try to explain previous events and why the
doctors did what they did. I'm not making excuses for
other doctors except to say that most of us do act in good
faith and try to do the best for our patients. I know that
sometimes, when I attempt to explain things to patients,
as hard as I try, they don't really hear my words because
the reality is just so painful to accept. What many people
do when they are upset about a situation is immediately
try to find something to blame it on. You can't be angry at
a disease, but you sure as hell can be angry at doctors,
nurses, and hospitals. One of the founders of hospice
(Elisabeth Kubler-Ross) said, "Blame it on God, He can
take it."

It's really difficult to accept that nothing more can be
done to fix this situation. In most cases, it is simply not
reasonable to begin more investigations, do more tests,
and attempt to place more stents. At some point one needs
to accept that no more interventions will materially help
the situation. He is unlikely to tolerate any procedures

and may very well be made worse, experience more dis-comfort, and die sooner. Many malignancies can progress and become symptomatic only when they have reached an advanced stage; a point at which cure is just not going to happen. It is often difficult for people to grasp how relentless some malignancies can be and how rapidly they produce a sudden decline when they have been develop-ing for some time. There seems to be little time to prepare when events like this happen so suddenly. No disease ever allows us enough time to adequately prepare.

#32 Incurable anger

> My husband Burt had cancer of the liver on top of cirrhosis. He was not a candidate for a new liver and did not do well with chemotherapy. When he became jaundiced and his belly swelled the oncologist sent him to have stents put in his liver. That helped for a while and then Burt got worse again. Our oncologist felt nothing additional would help him and referred us to hospice. I was told by another consultant at a big medical center that the stents were probably clogged. The hospice did not feel Burt would tolerate a long trip and the procedure. The hospice physician also explained that the quality of life would not improve and time left would not be much more. In fact, she said he might die sooner. I took him anyway and the doctor at the medical center did some studies, put in new stents and unclogged the old ones. I brought Burt home and two days later he died. I'm angry that new stents were not put in sooner to save my husband and don't think the hospice was aggressive enough. I know you don't exactly know Burt's case but I'm having trouble dealing with all of this.

You're correct about my not knowing every detail of Burt's illness, but I still can respond to your concerns because your situation, unfortunately, is not uncommon. I certainly hope that hospice was helpful at the end and that Burt's death was peaceful. You may not like all that I have to say but perhaps my words can provide some help. Your anger, I'm sure, is really about Burt's death and your grief about losing him. I need to continually remind myself that angry people are suffering. It's your suffering that needs to be addressed. Sometimes anger gets misdirected and serves no useful purpose. You could be angry with yourself for not listening to the hospice people and for subjecting your husband to a situation that may have brought death prematurely. There are a lot of places to direct your anger but that will change absolutely nothing except to keep stirring up the pot and prevent you from feeling what's underneath: sadness, grief, and feeling alone. Hospice can help you through this even though you did not heed their previous advice. You'd be advised to ask for their support and not be embarrassed because you did what you thought was the best thing to do. I'm sure your intention was to help and not to harm.

The hospice people and the medical center people also had good intentions. I suspect everyone did the best they could for Burt's incurable illness. One of the most frustrating emotions to experience is helplessness. Sometimes that feeling is intolerable. There is an urgency to do something—anything. Is that wrong? No. In retrospect, the situation might have been handled differently. Some might say you did the best you could do under the circumstances. There actually may be no correct answer but what's left now is this sense of incompleteness, the lack of resolution, and unfinished business. I'm sure you'll get through this and benefit from bereavement counseling. Please take this advice: ask for and get the support you need, allow your grief to lessen by itself as time passes, and get on with your life. I hope that advice helps.

#33 Sundowning

Mom has Alzheimer's dementia. For a long time she became more and more confused until we couldn't understand what she was saying. She was eating less and now spends most of her time in bed. She finally stopped talking and when she began to act really crazy in the evenings, the doctor put her on Haldol. She has some trouble swallowing and once in a while she will spit her food at us when we try to get her to eat. We tried to stop her Haldol and she just became very confused and restless. The hospice nurse restarted the medicine and then put in a urinary catheter so Mom wouldn't wet herself. The nurse thought maybe Mom was uncomfortable because she couldn't pass urine. I'm afraid to feed her because she might choke and anyway she really doesn't want to eat. If she doesn't eat, isn't she going to starve to death? Maybe she needs some IV fluids because she's getting dehydrated.

No one likes to sedate or tranquilize dying people unnecessarily. We do it to prevent them from injuring themselves and from suffering in a state of delirium. Delirium is a common event at the end of life. Some causes can be remedied, such as problems passing urine, moving bowels, or treating uncommunicated pain. Other causes may not be easily discovered and the agitation needs to be managed anyway. Spitting food is usually a signal that a person doesn't want to eat any longer. Eating and drinking naturally decline at the end of life. It is well recognized by those who treat the dying that the purpose of food at this stage is enjoyment, not nutrition. There is rarely value from forcing food or fluid. Patients can become congested (particularly if they receive fluids intravenously). Forcing feeding can cause people to choke or aspirate and can produce a great deal of suffering. In some cases, fluids can be given intravenously or subcutaneously but while it may temporarily clear some delirium, it does not always satisfy dry mouth. Good mouth care is about the best you can do. Words such as "dehydration" and "starvation" might apply to people who are able to recover from an illness and thrive. They are wrong and misleading terms to use here. Sometimes it's better to do nothing and support a natural dying process.

#34 Letting go

My wife is dying. Each time I walk into her room she seems weaker. I walk around feeling like crying most of the time. I don't want to worry her. I need to be the strong one because she depends on me. How am I supposed to let go?

You are letting go. Letting go doesn't happen all at once. It's a process that happens when you stay in your feelings. It has been said that the only way over something is by going through it. It seems paradoxical but you are strongest when you are brave enough to express and share your feelings. You can't skip the pain, because it is an integral part of the healing. I think the thing you miss seeing is the need for the sharing of your feelings. Crying with your wife and sharing the sadness is a sign of strength, not weakness. This is how she knows the depth of your feelings, and she will definitely benefit from doing her part to heal your pain in that sharing. Your wife is still the person she used to be on the inside. Her essence has not changed but your relationship is transforming. It's transcending form and the process of letting go becomes one of holding her differently. I don't think one ever lets go completely. You hold on with meaningful memories but without that cloud of grief enveloping you. That process simply takes its own time while life goes on.

#35 Dialysis and quality of life

Look at this picture of Harry. He looked so handsome in his army uniform when he was young. Now his doctor has referred him to hospice for his lung disease because he's always wheezing and needs medicine for his emphysema. On top of that he goes for dialysis three times a week and comes home more tired. He sleeps all the time and is not himself. Just look at him now. See how weak he is. He can hardly walk and is confused most of the time. I mean he's his old self some times and then he's back in lala land. The kidney specialist says he needs the dialysis or he won't last more than a few weeks. I can't just stop the dialysis and kill him. This isn't much of a life for me, is it? What am I supposed to do here? My kids say he has changed so much that he doesn't have much of a life being confused and sleeping all the time. I guess you see a lot of this, don't you?

Yes. Over the years, I've seen a lot of this and each time I need to remind myself that while it's not new for me, it's a unique, singular event for you. You know, when my father died in the intensive care unit of a large skilled nursing facility, I arrived after instructing them not to place him on a ventilator for life support if he did not recover from pneumonia. Of course, my dad was in an advanced stage of dementia and had no quality of life. When I walked into the intensive care unit, he was strapped down and intubated, on a ventilator. I simply walked over and pulled the plug. The nurse was horrified and said, "You can't do that." I replied, "I just did." The ventilator stopped and my father no longer breathed. He died quietly.

Looking back, I wonder how much of that action was to kill my pain and how much was to end his suffering.

Your husband is in a situation where his quality of life is diminishing. And by the way, so is yours. Looking out for yourself and your health is also an important factor in the decision. If you were to stop his dialysis, hospice could assist you in supporting his dying comfortably at home. I guess you need to ask yourself how much guilt you would suffer in the future having decided to terminate the dialysis. You certainly don't need to decide this alone and your family can help you establish at what point there is more harm than good in continuing dialysis. Just because a life-extending procedure is started does not mean that it cannot be stopped if it no longer is beneficial. Either way, it's important not to look back at some future time and question if you did the right thing or not.

I felt comfortable with my decision about my father because he no longer was the person I had known and had no quality of life as he would have defined it. I am not advocating impulsive behavior. In retrospect, I might have been a bit more diplomatic. That's in the past and it's over and I am certain that, under the circumstances, I did the best I could do. There will come a time when you no longer see the person you love in the same way you once did and you may justifiably decide to end his suffering. Letting go is a process and you need to trust yourself and your inner vision to recognize and accept when that time comes.

#36 A phone call

Hi, this is Dr. Appleton from hospice. Is this the Strickland residence? Is this Mr. Strickland?

Yes. What do you want?

I'm the hospice doctor and I'd like to come by and see Mrs. Strickland this morning if that's all right.

She's sleeping now. Can you come between 11:30 and 12:00?

Well, that's a little tight. Would there be a better time that would be a little more flexible?

You know, we just got on this damn hospice program and everybody's coming at once. My wife isn't that sick and besides she goes for her bridge club on Mondays, the church group on Tuesdays and Thursdays, and she gets her hair fixed on Fridays.

Would Wednesday be OK? I can be there between noon and four.

I guess that'll be OK. What are you going to do?

I thought I'd check her over and be sure everything is OK and that she's comfortable.

I'll see you on Wednesday, but be sure to call before you come.

It's not unusual for people to keep lists of activities, times for medications, records of bowel movements and schedules for everything. It's a way of feeling secure and in control. People are frequently afraid of making a mistake—particularly a fatal one. They require a lot of reassurance. Appointments for daily activities are important and a reminder for people that they are still alive. Even though these activities are small, they are meaningful and important. To interfere with these activities, particularly with unpleasant medical stuff, can be an intrusion and an admission of unwanted sickness and all that goes with it. While this may be viewed as a form of denial, it can also represent a healthy affirmation of life.

#37 Ending it all

My cancer is growing inside of me and I know I'm going to die. Even though I don't have a lot of pain I'm tired and feeling weak. Maybe I'm just depressed. Who wouldn' t be? I'm going to slug the next person who pats me on the shoulder and suggests I should cheer up a little and enjoy the life I've got left. It's easy to give advice if you don't have what I've got and yet here I am asking for your advice. Truthfully, I'd just like this to be over with and quit this waiting game. Maybe you can give me something to knock me out and end this.

I hear you. It's impossible for me to know how you feel. Yes, it sounds as if you're depressed and a pat on the shoulder will do nothing but drive you further into sadness. No one should expect you to be upbeat about your situation and I guess I'd ask you what it would take, short of ending your life prematurely, to make your remaining life worth living. Depression and the sense of being helplessly alone can feel like a whirlpool sucking you deeper into its depths. I think a possible way out is to reach out for a human connection to help extract you from the vortex or whatever seems to be pulling you deeper into despair. It won't change the situation but it might change the angst. Perhaps it will be helpful if I tell you a short story. Please understand that I am not discounting your feelings or your situation.

I had a good friend who was dying of liver cancer and who actually tried, unsuccessfully, to overdose on pain medicine. He had talked about how difficult it was for him to go through this interminable wait for his life to end. I can imagine that using medication to have some control and to kill the emotional pain of waiting looked like a good way out. We found him in a stupor and really thought it was the end. Then he rallied and was his old self again the next day. He denied taking an overdose but began talking to me about feeling alone and angry and depressed. He said he'd been thinking a lot about suicide. I did not tell him I knew about his failed attempt.

Let me share with you what I told him and see if any of this is of any benefit to you. "You know that suicide is not the answer. It's an angry act that solves nothing well and inflicts pain on those you leave behind. They'll always wonder what they could have done to help and why you chose anger and loneliness to push them away instead of reaching out to include them. I can't tell you how to get out of your doldrums. That's why I'm here. I may be only a momentary distraction, but as your friend I need to feel less powerless in helping both of us out of this sad place. Does that make sense? I know this sounds off-the-wall, but maybe we can do something really dumb and outrageous to blow away this black cloud. I know! Do you like candy bars? How about if I run out to the market and buy some candy like Snickers, Mars bars, and a lot of junk like that?"

He said he liked Peppermint Patties. I thought to myself it might sweeten his sour mood but didn't say that. So I left and returned with twenty dollars worth of assorted candy, which we proceeded to dump onto the coffee table and consume like greedy little kids at Halloween. Now I know this sounds silly, and believe me, I am not making light of your situation. I just know that finding some other person to help you climb out of your pit and back into another moment of life is one way to help. Maybe you can get creative. You are not dead yet so perhaps you can think outside of the box. At worst it will be a waste of time, but you're doing that anyway. It turns out that my friend lived another month before he died, and in that period experienced some wonderful times, which we all enjoyed sharing with him.

#38 Tapping the fluid

Charley has lung cancer. He is short of breath and needs oxygen all the time. When he was in the hospital the doctor took fluid off of his lung. They said they got a lot and it helped his breathing for a while. Why can't that be done again?

This is a difficult problem and although it seems simple to pull some fluid off, it's a very short period until the fluid returns. We see this in ascites (where fluid fills the abdominal cavity) and in chest diseases like Charley's. Tubes can be placed to provide a continuous drainage into an outside collection bag. These frequently get plugged and need to be replaced. There are some methods of injecting substances into the chest cavity to stop the fluid accumulation. This is usually uncomfortable and not always successful. There are other complications with repeat draining of fluid, such as infection and bleeding, and eventually (usually within a period of weeks) draining the fluid becomes impossible. Taking off large volumes of fluid can also cause marked fluid shifts within the body and can actually accelerate the process of dying. Certainly there are times when another tap might be used to extend life for a meaningful life event such as a birth or a wedding, but eventually all methods of removing fluid fail as disease progresses. Difficulty breathing can be relieved with medication and death can usually be made peaceful.

#39 Drugs and more drugs

> My wife was doing fine on her medicines before she got sick and dragged off to the hospital. She was on about ten different pills, which cost a lot of money. Now she's back home with another bunch of pills, different from what she had before. I just don't get this and I'd like to chuck the whole lot. I know they found cancer of her ovary and she ain't gonna live too long. How am I supposed to figure this stuff out? Can you explain that?

I know drugs are expensive and their names confusing. There are different names for similar drugs—some are labeled as generic and others, which may be the same drug, have a different trade name. It's even confusing for those of us who prescribe medicine to keep the names straight. If a patient sees several doctors, each doctor will prescribe his/her favorite specialty drug and pretty soon the poor patient has such a pot-full of drugs, some of which may be duplicates, that it really is almost impossible to know which drug to take and when to take it. I sometimes wonder how people have room for food in their stomachs with all the pills. If there is a side effect, it's a guessing game to pick the offending pill. I understand how frustrating this whole thing is, particularly when you are worried about your wife. Imagine how difficult it would be for her to figure out the drugs when she's not feeling well if you weren't there to help.

Let me offer some suggestions. I don't know every drug your wife has had prescribed for her and I don't know her other conditions. I do know that when there are more than five drugs on the list, we already have a probability of drug-drug interactions and more potential problems.

First, it helps to have help from one doctor and your hospice nurse—you do not need to do this alone, so just relax. Second, sort the drugs by the different conditions or the specialty of the doctor who prescribed the medication. Spread the bottles out on the dining room table. Next, get rid of any over-the-counter drugs, aspirin, cold remedies, laxatives, etc. Don't worry: we won't let your wife get constipated. Now I'd get rid of cholesterol drugs for the time being. It usually won't hurt to hold off vitamins and thyroid for a few days. You can always add back in hormones like thyroid or estrogen at a later date. The idea here is to keep cardiac medications and other necessary drugs and eliminate non-essential medications. We can help with that. What is important in the hospice program is to treat your wife's pain and the symptoms associated with her cancer. Those will be the primary drugs to employ. Then we can slowly go through necessary and unnecessary drugs for the present situation.

I suspect that the drugs your wife was taking before she went to the hospital were correct and now that her situation has changed, it makes sense to prioritize what are the current basic drugs required. As an example, if your wife was on oral diabetic medications, has lost weight, and is eating less, perhaps she does not require the same diabetic regimen. All of this can be straightened out. Don't panic. Let's make a list, write down the names of the drugs, and match the drugs to the conditions. Then we can pick the ones to use and the ones to set aside. After that we can make a comfortable schedule to fit your lifestyle. This whole program, even though it is new to you, is to make life easier to enjoy without feeling glued to the pillbox.

I want to offer one other thought now that we're starting to get a handle on the pill problem. You sounded angry when you asked your question. I know this whole thing can make a person feel out of control and your difficult situation can really set you off. I know from my own experience that the thing about which I'm angry is not the real reason; it's just the most convenient outlet and just the tip of my iceberg. I'm not being critical and I know there will be other times when you'll get irritated. If you can just recognize when you begin to sizzle you might take a deep breath and know the upset is really about what's going on with your wife's illness and not the particular event that set you off. This is a tough situation and with each event you can stop for a moment, choose the best response, and be gentle with everyone, including yourself.

#40 New is not always better

Our mother has breast cancer. When she first discovered a lump in her breast she was frightened about what it might be and she waited to see if it would go away. It didn't go away. When the tumor of the breast got larger she hid it under large dresses and was embarrassed to go to the doctor because she felt stupid. When the cancer became painful, broke through the skin, and was draining we finally got her to a doctor who said it was too late for surgery, and she had to go into a hospice program. She heard about a clinic in Mexico where they promise to cure cancer. They use special diets and treatments that are not used in the United States. My mother is from Mexico and wants to try this treatment in her country but my sisters and I worry that maybe we should try to do something here first.

I don't know enough about the extent of your mother's cancer. She needs to see an oncologist, have a biopsy, and have all her options explained clearly. Then she can choose. If she chooses no hormone therapy, no chemotherapy, or no radiation then hospice is a choice. She can also have these cancer treatments, if they are acceptable to her and her cancer does not progress too far. She can be cared for by hospice afterwards if cure is not possible. My experience with cancer clinics south of the border has been dismal. I am sure there are well-trained cancer specialists in Mexico, however I am very suspicious of places that offer cures with diet, coffee enemas, and less than scientific detoxification remedies for cancer and other ailments. They may have some placebo effect, particularly if they're costly, but you need to wonder why these treatments are not offered north of the border. I personally do not believe that there is a conspiracy by the medical establishment to keep these treatments out of the United States. The laws are designed to protect innocent people from being victimized by unproven treatments and fraudulent claims. The bottom line here is to get an opinion from one or more reputable specialists here and then, if you still decide to travel south, please be cautious.

#41 Sudden change/sudden impact

Mom was walking around last week: we were playing Scrabble and watching TV. She had a headache and became confused. We went to the emergency room where we waited four hours. Finally, this doctor came into the waiting room and told us Mom had brain cancer and was going to die. Just like that. He said he was sending us to a hospice program and putting her in a nursing home. Then he just walked out. We were in shock and the next thing we knew, some hospice people showed up to sign us up and sign a bunch of papers. This all happened so fast and was so confusing we really didn't know what to do. When I got angry with the way we had been treated, nobody really listened or helped us to figure out what was going on.

It's impossible to imagine the impact of sudden change in a loved one and horrible bad news about their condition unless you've been through it yourself. It's difficult enough to see a loved one deteriorate slowly from a terminal illness but at least there is usually some time to prepare. I don't think there is a word to describe the sense of overwhelm you must have experienced. I'm sure rapid change from "alive and well" to "going to die" clouds your ability to hear any explanations when you are in that state of shock. Being hurried out of the hospital into a hospice program without sensitivity and a gentle transition is enough to cause anybody to flare. Sometimes there is just no way to deliver bad news without inflicting pain, however a transition to hospice in a supportive and caring manner can certainly cushion the impact and modify an experience such as yours.

One of the difficult problems we encounter when families are faced with the sudden decline of a loved one is helping people adjust to the progressive disease process. Perhaps it will help to understand that frequently symptoms are just the tip of the iceberg. The underlying disease may have been present for some time when suddenly uncontrollable symptoms appear. It is then that the patient is taken to the emergency room, studied, and perhaps treated. Often when an untreatable or terminal disease is diagnosed at this point, the patient is referred to hospice for end-of-life care. This comes as an unexpected shock.

Angry patients and families demand to know why the disease was not found earlier. The anger also spills over to blaming the rapid changes on medications given for pain rather than appreciating the real cause—a disease that is now presenting itself with many more apparent symptoms.

Having said that, and I'm not condoning the insensitive behavior that you perceived on the part of the physician, I really think you need to move past what happened and see what can be done for Mom and the entire family now. Staying focused now is where you are going to be most effective, not rehashing thoughtless behavior and holding on to anger. Hopefully, hospice can help you manage your mother now, whether it is at home or a nursing facility. There is a lot happening, which is confusing. Try to maintain a non-anxious presence. The focus here is on Mom's comfort at the end of her life and your quality time spent with her now.

I hate platitudes because they offer a sugar coating and often seem to minimize one's experience. Anyway, here is a thought to carry with you. It is not an excuse for unfortunate and painful life events as much as a way to personally move away from anger and regret and disappointment. I think it is at the core of moving more productively through this transition. It's about forgiveness; forgiving the imperfections in the medical system, medicine, and the people who practice it; forgiving insensitivity and not taking it personally; forgiving your loved one for abandoning you; and finally, forgiving yourself for expressions of upset and for irrational behavior.

Sometimes we're really hard on ourselves and unforgiving of our own imperfections. There is something about forgiving that helps relieve some of the hurt and allows you to stay focused in the present moment.

#42 Knock me out

When my sister was dying of breast cancer the doctors couldn't stop her pain. They kept pumping her full of more and more morphine and nothing seemed to work. The hospice physician suggested palliative sedation and then they started some intravenous drugs that kept her unconscious until she passed away. Was that the right thing to do?

From my standpoint, it would have been wrong to allow your sister to be in pain until the end. Ideally, one would prefer a person to be awake and pain-free until death. There are times when that's just not possible, and if comfort at the end of life is only possible with a state of unconsciousness, then palliative terminal sedation is the answer. I would like to think we can stop physical pain in order to be able to deal with the emotional and spiritual pain of dying and sometimes the ideal situation is impossible to achieve. She was not sedated because you or your family couldn't bear her pain and wanted it over for your sake. I'm not suggesting that your suffering was unimportant but the primary focus was on helping your sister and she was sedated for her sake to allow a peaceful death.

#43 Do everything

Hello doctor, this is Mrs. Veerbose, I'm Olga Swarb's daughter. Do you remember my mother? You were at the house six months ago when mom was diagnosed with cancer and given two months to live. Now do you remember?

Yes. It's been a while but I do recall the visit. How is your mother doing and what can I do for you?

My mother has a swollen ankle and I want an X-ray immediately to see if it's broken.

Has your mother been walking?

Of course not! Don't you remember she never walked after her stroke?

So she's bed-bound. Was our hospice nurse over to see her?

Oh sure! But she said to just wrap it and I don't think that's good enough. Just last week I got her to the emergency room for her cough and they gave her antibiotics. The hospice nurse said cough medicine was enough. Just because she's on hospice we can't just let her die. What would you do if it were your mother?

Hold on for a moment and let me ask a few questions to refresh my memory. Can your mother talk and is she eating?

Of course not! She was never able to talk or swallow after the stroke and that's when they put that tube into her stomach for feeding. Do you remember now?

Yes, yes. I remember. Let me see if I've got this straight. Your mother has cancer and has lived longer that predicted. She's had a stroke and cannot speak or eat and you feed her through a gastrostomy. Is that correct?

Yes, that's what I just told you!

I understand that's what you just told me. What I have trouble understanding is why you want to continue emergency visits when the purpose of hospice is not to cure every medical problem that arises but to keep your mother comfortable at the end of her life. I don't think we are being neglectful by avoiding emergency rooms. I think we are being practical. We're treating a cough without throwing antibiotics at her and I frankly don't see the value of an X-ray if your mother is not walking—we're probably not going to put the foot in a cast.

Look, doctor! This is my mother and I want to do the right thing. Do you understand?

Mrs. Veerbose. I understand completely. You asked me before what I'd do if this were my mother so let me tell you. I'd be concerned also about getting things right and not making a mistake. I'd also realize that my mom is at the end of life and not everything can be fixed. I know that as soon as you fix one thing another pops up, which, by the way, may be worse than the one you just fixed. Please listen to me. You and I both know that your mother is dying and that this is difficult for you to deal with. The hardest thing to do is nothing. In your situation, nothing may be the best choice. You cannot fix your mom and believe me; if you let us help to keep her comfortable, that's enough.

Before I hang up, I need to be straightforward with you and hope you'll listen carefully to my words. My

81

intention is to make this situation better for both you and your mother. Things will go better if you can make a change in the way you present your concerns. There is something in the way you express yourself that feels like an attack. I don't think that's what you mean, but it makes me want to run. While I may understand that this is a painful experience for you, not everybody will be receptive to your needs if they come across as demands. You should understand that people who feel shamed or become defensive by your attitude may be put off. We would like to be gentle and supportive and we hope you'll allow us help both you and your mother.

#44 Morpheus—god of dreams

Dad's doctor referred him to a hospice program. He has heart failure, and was short of breath and on a lot of medications. The day he was put on hospice he was alert but had some pain and they gave him a half-dropper of morphine under his tongue. He fell asleep after one dose and now he is sleeping all the time and is hard to awaken. It's been two days now and he just lies there. Are they trying to kill him with the morphine or what?

I doubt the hospice people are trying to kill your dad. That's just not what hospice is about. You bring up a rather common problem, which I'll try to explain. Having a terminal illness is a tremendous stress on the body and most people in your dad's situation are fatigued—particularly with heart failure. The amount of morphine in dropper form that was given was probably about 10 milligrams—that's a pretty low dose. It is unlikely that the morphine caused the sudden change in your dad's condition. Sure, it would make him rest, but his rapid decline is more likely the result of his end-stage disease rather than the morphine. When families see a sudden change in a loved one's condition, it's usually easier to blame some medicine rather than accept the end-stage disease as the cause of the decline. That's not to say that medications never contribute to what appears to be a worsening of a condition. It's usually very difficult to accept just how close the end really is. I hope the hospice people have been able to help.

That does bring up another thought, which I can share with you. There are a lot of myths about morphine, which condition a person's thinking about the drug. I am sometimes reluctant to even use the "M" word because there are so many misconceptions about morphine. It's a good drug with a few side effects. Using it does not mean the end is near or things are necessarily getting worse. When I suspect a patient or family is fearful, I avoid doing battle and simply use an alternative drug. Even then, it's often the drugs that get blamed first rather than the disease progression, which is more difficult to accept.

#45 An ending

My wife slipped into a coma. Her breathing was regular but she seemed a little congested. I gave her some drops under her tongue and it seemed to dry up the airway. I thought it might be near the end and I didn't know what else to do. I climbed onto the hospital bed with her, lay down next to her, and put my head on her chest. I guess I must have fallen asleep. When I opened my eyes it was very quiet. She had stopped breathing and had died. I don't know if that was the right thing to do or if I could have done anything else.

What a wonderful and peaceful end. You did well.

#46 When to stop

Stanley and I have been married for forty-two years. He has been on dialysis for a year and recently the emergency room doctor said that he was coming into the hospital too often for his bad emphysema attacks. He said we ought to go on a hospice program. Stan felt that was a good idea because he hated being short of breath and getting tubes shoved down him every time his breathing got bad. We are on hospice now and the nurses come to the house. One of the nurses asked why Stanley was still going for dialysis three times a week. I know he doesn't like to spend his days there and sometimes he gets kind of confused. In the middle of dialysis he pleads with me to just take him home. He is so weak and short of breath and sleeps most of the time he is at home. I know this isn't much of a life, but I can't just stop the dialysis treatments, can I? If he stops dialysis he will die. I feel like I'd be killing him.

I doubt that it will help to tell you that your situation is not at all uncommon. Hospice is about helping people to live as fully as possible. It's about squeezing the most quality of life out of the time left. Sometimes life reaches a state where it is just not worth living the way it is. I think the important thing here is not to diminish life's quality by trips for dialysis, blood tests, shunt revisions, and other procedures. If Stanley gets confused and does not want to continue dialysis, I would respect his wishes. It is his life and his decision if he wishes to stop. I know letting go is difficult, but why keep him alive longer so that he can suffer more? Stopping dialysis is not the same as killing him. It's allowing him to end his life comfortably. I see it as a loving gift. The end of life for people dying in renal failure is usually not uncomfortable.

#47 The need to know

Look, doctor! It's as simple as this. Daddy doesn't need to know he has cancer. He doesn't know he's dying and we don't want you to tell him. My mom and I think it'll kill him if he knows; he'll just give up. I mean, he knows he's sick but we don't want him to give up hope. Mom said he was talking yesterday about all his friends who died. I think it's all the drugs he's taking. Can't we just keep treating him without letting on this is the end? His main concern is why he feels so weak and tired. He wants to know when he's going to get better. Maybe you could tell him we're working on it.

If I speak with your father, I don't need to bring up his cancer in the beginning, but if he asks, I won't lie. Some people know they are dying and simply avoid talking about it. Denial is interesting in that it is a way people automatically shield themselves from an uncomfortable reality until they can incorporate it into their personal reality. Some people never do and need to remain defended from the emotional pain. Denial applies to you also—not telling dad may be your way of not having to face his reaction to being told. I'm not making you wrong, I'm only trying to help you through this situation and explain your responses. The fact that he mentioned his friends dying indicates to me that somewhere inside he really does know what's going on. If you ask him if he knows what's going on and if he wants to know even if it's bad news, watch his response. If he says yes, tell him he has cancer and that hospice will help him get through this even though there isn't a cure. If he becomes evasive, looks away, changes the subject, or avoids your question, I suspect he knows and at the same time does not want to know. Then leave it alone. He's probably weak and fatigued from his disease, although his medications can also have some side effects.

As far as people giving up hope when they hear they have a terminal disease, I personally have not experienced that. It's true that some depression may appear. That's a normal reaction, but most people don't stay permanently depressed, particularly if they receive support from family and hospice. I've said before that the nature of hope changes and there can still be some meaningful life experiences left to enjoy. What bothers me about not telling the truth is not just that is covert lying but that, by not being forthright, we create a state of emotional isolation for the patient. Please read Emily Dickenson's poem at the beginning of this book again. I know this is a difficult and painful situation for you and your parents. There is no absolutely correct way to manage this problem and there is no way to predict responses. What I know is that it takes courage to move through this process. I'm sure you have that. Let your heart lead you along your path.

#48 Gathering at the end

I saw you getting out of your car yesterday as I was driving by those run-down apartments near my house. I saw you going into that apartment where that crowd of Mexican people were hanging around. I figured that it must have been bad like a shooting or something if you were making a house call.

It's interesting that you should think that. Actually, I was making a home visit to a dying woman. I went to see her and talk to her family. All of those people you saw were family and a few friends. It is a wonderful tradition in Latino culture for the families to gather when someone is dying. If you think it was crowded outside you should have been inside. The place was packed. I have never been treated with so much respect and reverence as I was at that visit. There were babies crying and small children running around and people sitting everywhere; talking, crying, eating and taking turns talking to my patient at her bedside. There was certainly a lot of sadness there but also there seemed to be a natural acceptance of the end of life. It really made me proud to be included and be able to support the family by answering their questions and doing my best to allay their fears. The involvement of extended family and friends is an age-old tradition in many cultures. I have tremendous respect for this traditional gathering of families and the involvement of all ages as witness to dying.

#49 Emotional cutoff

> My husband died in a hospice program. One day he
> was playing golf and the next day he had a stroke and
> went into a coma. The doctor said nothing more could
> be done and he should be in a hospice program. I
> took him home and cared for him for a week before
> he died. Hospice really helped. They were great
> except for that dumb nurse who kept patting me on
> the shoulder when I was crying and telling me, "I
> know just how you feel, dear."
>
> Now he's dead and I'm going to get rid of his stuff.
> I'm going to put pictures away and move on. Funny
> thing is that sometimes I see a shadow in the
> bathroom and think I see him shaving, but he's not
> there. How long is that going to go on?

Sudden death doesn't give you much chance to
prepare. Having had time to adjust before the death of
your husband may have cushioned the blow some, but it's
a terrible loss nonetheless. It's going to take a while to
adjust to the loss. A large piece of your life and your
history is gone. This is not a good time to make major decisions. Disposing of your husband's belongings prematurely to make the pain go away probably is not a good
idea in the long run. It is really healing to look through old
things and recall past events that hopefully were joyful.
Wait a while. It can take a while to regroup and redefine
yourself after this loss. The hospice bereavement people
are wonderful counselors and can be of tremendous help
in getting you through. As far as that nurse was concerned,
I guess it was her way of trying to help, but that's just the
wrong behavior. She had no way of actually being inside
you and knowing how you felt. It would have been best if
she'd kept her mouth closed. As for that gratuitous pat on

the shoulder, we call that a band-aid. It is an unconscious attempt to shut you up to keep herself from getting to close to your pain. She's got some personal work to do and you probably shouldn't take her misguided attempt personally. As for thinking you saw your husband shaving, it's not uncommon for a surviving partner to have flashes as if the spouse was still there. That's a part of the adjustment process. When fleeting moments like that do occur, it might be an opportunity for you to stop what you're doing and have a conversation with your husband as if he were actually there. He will always be there as a part of your memory, but you'll embrace the thoughts in a different way.

#50 Recollection and appreciation

As I look back on the past few months it seems almost unreal. So much happened so fast and I've never been through such a flood of feelings. When my husband came home from the doctor's office at the beginning of this his face was ashen. Our family physician sent him for a consultation with an oncologist but didn't seem too concerned. In retrospect, I think he didn't want to frighten us prematurely. I didn't even go with John for the appointment because it seemed so routine. I knew John had a lot of tests done but he never had much to say about them. I just figured that no news was good news. So when he came home looking like a ghost I got worried and then he dropped the bomb that he had widespread incurable cancer with less than six months to live. To make a long story short, we got a second opinion, which confirmed the diagnosis. The second doctor even said that a biopsy wasn't necessary because it did not matter what type of cancer it was since there was no available treatment and besides, John was too far gone to benefit from any treatment. Then the second doctor called our family doctor and then we were referred to hospice. In the beginning, John didn't have any pain but as he got weaker and lost more weight he began to have more and more pain. The hospice specialist got that under control quickly, although I was pretty shaken up when morphine arrived (but it worked great).

What I want to tell you is that we went from feeling totally lost and defeated to feeling supported and cared for by the hospice people. They explained a lot to us but in the beginning I don't think we heard much. We were so confused and upset. I know I was pretty angry about this happening and I wondered why the cancer wasn't caught sooner. John just kind of closed down for a while and I seemed to be the crazy one, crying one minute and screaming on the phone the next. It took a while to settle down and eventually we got to know the hospice nurses and the home health aides. He even let them bathe him when he couldn't get out of bed. I liked the doctor a lot and the counselors were wonderful. We got to work through a lot of problems and get through a lot of stuff. Even the bereavement people were great.

I guess the reason I'm telling you this is because more people should know about what you do and how you really make a contribution to people at the end of life. When John died in his sleep the hospice nurse came out and hospice arranged everything; they even had their chaplain perform the funeral ceremony. This was one of the most difficult experiences of my life. When I look back I have fond memories of the wonderful people who gave us so much love. When I look at the night sky I see my John in all the stars.

"Give me my Romeo; and, when he shall die,
Take him and cut him out in little stars,
And he will make the face of heaven so fine
That all the world will be in love with night,
And pay no worship to the garish sun."

—William Shakespeare, *Romeo and Juliet*

About the author

Michael Appleton is an internist specializing in hospice and palliative care. He is board certified in addiction medicine and in hospice and palliative medicine. As the medical director of Odyssey Healthcare in Rancho Mirage, California, he continues to make home visits to terminally ill patients.

Printed in the United States
70163LV00002B/61

9 781587 364815